HYDROGEN MEDICINE GUIDE FOR ADULTS.

Nancy S Brooks

2.3. Impact on Cardiovascular Health

2.4. Neuroprotective Benefits

2.5. Detoxification and Immune system Support.

CHAPTER 3. APPLICATIONS AND PRACTICES OF HYDROGEN MEDICINE

3.1. Inhalation Therapy: Breathing Hydrogen Gas

3.2. Hydrogen-Enriched Water and Beverages

CONCLUSION

CHAPTER 1. INTRODUCTION TO HYDROGEN MEDICINE

1.1. Background and History.

Hydrogen has been used in medicine for centuries, a remarkably lengthy and fascinating history. Recent scientific developments have rekindled enthusiasm for its potential as a medicinal agent, despite its history being characterized by periods of great interest followed by relative obscurity. Take a peek at the intriguing history of adult hydrogen medicine:

The first indications of hydrogen's use in medicine date back to James Watt and Thomas Beddoes' research in the eighteenth century. In order to treat diseases like tuberculosis and asthma, they experimented with inhaling several gases, including hydrogen.

The 19th century saw the investigation of molecular hydrogen's potential for internal wound localization. In order to prove the existence of gastrointestinal tract punctures, rectal insufflation of hydrogen gas paved the way for potentially life-saving procedures.

The medicinal qualities of hydrogen experienced a rise in interest in the early 20th century. It was applied in a variety of ways, including the treatment of burns, enhancing sports performance, and even combating cancer. But by the middle of the 20th century, enthusiasm had begun to fade due to uneven findings and methodological problems in the research.

Current research indicates that molecular hydrogen can function as a selective antioxidant, focusing on harmful free radicals while sparing beneficial ones, and may have applications in treating a range of medical conditions. These findings have rekindled interest in hydrogen medicine. Molecular hydrogen can be inhaled or consumed as hydrogen-enriched water.

The antioxidant and anti-inflammatory qualities of hydrogen may be beneficial for treating neurological illnesses like Parkinson's and Alzheimer's. According to preliminary research, it may preserve brain tissue and enhance cognitive performance.

One possible use for hydrogen is in the treatment of chronic inflammatory diseases including pain and arthritis because of its capacity to lower oxidative stress and inflammation.

The protective properties of hydrogen may help tissues after surgery or organ transplantation by reducing harm during blood flow restoration.

Although hydrogen medicine has a lot of potential, it's vital to keep in mind that research is still in its infancy. Further high-quality clinical trials are required to confirm its safety and effectiveness in different adult populations. Furthermore, additional research is needed to determine the best delivery strategies and dosing guidelines.

Adult hydrogen medicine has a fascinating and promising history that alternates between moments of fervor and doubt. It's encouraging that interest is currently reviving due to exciting new studies. However, before hydrogen is extensively used as a medicinal agent, careful and thorough scientific research is required. If this medieval substance can truly change modern adult medicine, only time will tell.

1.2. Molecular Hydrogen and it's Therapeutic potential

The simplest molecule in the universe is called molecular hydrogen (H_2), which is made up of simply two protons joined by a single electron. However, don't undervalue its capabilities! According to recent studies, H_2 has exceptional therapeutic characteristics that provide promise for treating a variety of adult health issues.

H2's capacity to function as a selective antioxidant is one of its main advantages. H_2 specifically scavenges the dangerous hydroxyl radical (OH·), a highly reactive molecule linked to a number of disorders, in contrast to conventional antioxidants that target both good and bad free radicals. This focused strategy counteracts the harmful effects of oxidative stress while assisting in the protection of healthy cells.

Moreover, H2 has strong anti-inflammatory qualities. By modifying the immune system's reaction, it lowers the generation of mediators of inflammation such as chemokines and cytokines. This may help with ailments like arthritis, persistent pain, and even neurological illnesses by reducing the chain reaction of inflammation.

Several medical specialties are actively investigating H_2's medicinal potential. The anti-inflammatory and antioxidant characteristics of H_2 may be able to shield brain tissue and slow the advancement of neurodegenerative illnesses like Parkinson's and Alzheimer's. According to preliminary research, patients' memory and cognitive performance may improve. When blood flow is restored after a period of deprivation, tissues may sustain injury during surgery or organ transplantation. The preventive actions of H_2 may reduce this damage, improving patient outcomes. Metabolic illnesses such as obesity and diabetes are characterized by oxidative stress and chronic inflammation. The potential benefits of H_2 in managing these disorders and enhancing general metabolic health are suggested by its ability to counteract these effects.

There are several ways to deliver molecular hydrogen, which includes; Inhaling gas mixes or air that has been enhanced with H2O, Water that is high in hydrogen, and Intravenous injection for precise, focused delivery.

1.3. Overview of Hydrogen Medicine Research

In the field of medicine, molecular hydrogen (H_2), the most basic chemical in the universe, is showing great promise. Research on its therapeutic uses for a range of medical problems has exploded due to its ability to fight inflammation and oxidative damage. Now let's explore the exciting field of hydrogen medicine research:

As a selective antioxidant, H_2 destroys dangerous hydroxyl radicals (OH·) but spares healthy free radicals. This focused strategy aids in shielding healthy cells from oxidative damage, which is a major cause of numerous illnesses.

Due to its anti-inflammatory qualities, H_2 helps control the immune system's reaction by lowering the synthesis of inflammatory mediators. It may therefore be an ally in the treatment of ailments like neurodegenerative disorders, chronic pain, and arthritis.

Researchers are now investigating the possibilities of H_2 in a number of fields like:

- **Neurodegenerative Diseases:** According to research, people with Parkinson's and Alzheimer's disease may benefit from increased cognitive performance and brain cell protection with H3.

- **Ischemia-Reperfusion Injury:** By reducing tissue damage after surgery or organ transplantation, H_2 may have a protective impact.

- **Metabolic Diseases:** By reducing inflammation and oxidative stress, H_2 may be able to help control diabetes and obesity.

The research on H_2 therapy is still in its early phases, despite the encouraging results. Further extensive clinical trials are required to validate its effectiveness and safety in various circumstances. Additional research is needed to determine the ideal dosage and administration methods.

The potential of H_2 treatment is evident despite the difficulties. Because of its special qualities, it presents a fresh way to address a range of health problems, opening the door for this old molecule to one day be an important instrument in our

medical toolbox

CHAPTER 2. HEALTH BENEFITS OF MOLECULAR HYDROGEN

2.1 Antioxidant Properties and Cellular Health

The fundamental components of life, our cells are always trying to keep us alive and functioning. However, dangerous substances known as free radicals are always attacking them, just like any other machine. These substances are extremely reactive and can harm cells, which can result in a number of health issues.

Antioxidants are thankfully our bodies' built-in defense mechanism against free radicals. Similar to scavengers, these molecules locate free radicals and neutralize them before they have a chance to do any harm.

The following are some ways that antioxidant qualities support cellular health:

- Combating Free Radicals: Consider free radicals as microscopic bullies destroying your cells. Like super heroes, antioxidants intervene to neutralize these bullies and stop

them from doing any damage. As a
result, there is less oxidative stress,
which is linked to chronic illnesses
and aging.

- DNA protection: Our cells' genetic
  code, the DNA, can be harmed by
  free radicals. Mutations and even
  cancer may result from this.
  Antioxidants assist in defending our
  DNA from these assaults,
  maintaining the health and efficiency
  of our cells.

- Increasing Immunity: Antioxidants
  are essential for maintaining our
  defenses against disease. They
  support the immune cells that defend

our body against infections and other dangers, preserving our health and averting illness.

- Minimizing Inflammation: While inflammation is a normal reaction to trauma or infection, prolonged inflammation can harm internal organs and tissues. Since antioxidants have anti-inflammatory qualities, they aid in reducing inflammation and shielding our cells from more harm.
- Supporting Repair and Regeneration: Antioxidants aid in the stimulation of damaged cells' ability to repair and regenerate. Maintaining the health of

the body's tissues and organs
depends on this.

The good news is that a diet rich in
antioxidants is within reach. These are a
few of the top resources:

- Fruits and vegetables: Rich sources
  of antioxidants include peppers,
  citrus fruits, leafy greens, and
  berries. To reap the greatest
  spectrum of antioxidant advantages,
  aim for a diversity of colors.
- Nuts and seeds: Rich sources of
  antioxidants include walnuts,
  almonds, chia seeds, and flaxseeds.

- Whole grains: Oats, quinoa, and brown rice are examples of whole grains that are rich in antioxidants.
- Fish: Omega-3 fatty acids are abundant in fatty fish, such as mackerel, salmon, and tuna, and they have antioxidant qualities.
- Dark chocolate: Dark chocolate with at least 70% cocoa content is a good source of antioxidants.

In addition to diet, there are other ways to boost your antioxidant levels, which includes;

- Exercise regularly: Exercise helps to increase your body's natural production of antioxidants.

- Get enough sleep: Sleep deprivation can reduce your body's antioxidant levels.

- Chocolate that is dark: Dark chocolate that has at least 70% cocoa is an excellent source of antioxidants.

However, there are further methods to increase your antioxidant levels outside diet:

- Engage in regular exercise: Exercise promotes the body's natural synthesis of antioxidants.

- Obtain adequate rest; insufficient sleep lowers the levels of antioxidants in your body.

- Manage your stress: Antioxidants can be depleted by stress. Take up yoga, meditation, or time spent in nature as beneficial stress-reduction techniques.

Your cells will be well-protected against the harmful effects of free radicals and will continue to function normally for many years if you adopt these lifestyle changes.

The greatest strategies to ensure that your body gets the antioxidants it needs are to maintain a balanced diet and lifestyle. It's advisable to see your doctor before starting any new supplement regimen, even if vitamins might be beneficial in certain situations.

2.2 Anti-inflammatory Effects on the Body

Our body's immunological response naturally includes inflammation. This defense mechanism aids in the healing of injured tissue and the prevention of infection. Chronic inflammation, on the other hand, can be harmful and cause a number of conditions, including cancer, heart disease, and arthritis.

The Mechanism of Inflammation are as follows;

- Injury or Infection: Your body
  releases white blood cells to the site
  of injury when it senses a threat,
  such as a cut or a virus.

- Chemical Release: These white
  blood cells secrete substances known
  as inflammatory mediators, which
  include cytokines and
  prostaglandins.

- Increased Blood Flow: As the blood
  vessels in the region enlarge, more
  fluids and white blood cells can get
  to the injured area.

- Pain and Swelling: Pain, redness,
  warmth, and swelling are brought on

by the accumulation of fluid and increased blood flow.

Moreover, there are Inflammatory agents which are drugs that aid in lowering inflammation and the symptoms that go along with it. They operate differently based on the type. Aspirin, ibuprofen, and naproxen are examples of nonsteroidal anti-inflammatory drugs (NSAIDs), which are the most widely used class of anti-inflammatory medications. They function by preventing the synthesis of the following:

- prostaglandins, which are molecules that aggravate pain and inflammation.

- Corticosteroids: These are potent topical, oral, or injectable anti-inflammatory medications. They function by reducing the inflammatory response of the immune system.

- Biological agents are more recent medications that concentrate on particular pathways involved in inflammation. Their application is common in the management of long-term inflammatory diseases such as

Crohn's disease and rheumatoid arthritis.

There are body's anti-inflammatory effects like:

- Decreased Swelling: Anti-inflammatories work to lessen the amount of fluid that accumulates in the injured area, which helps to ease pain and swelling.
- Pain Relief: Anti-inflammatories have the ability to significantly reduce inflammation and block pain signals.

- Enhanced Mobility: You may be able to move about more easily and have a greater range of motion if you have less discomfort and edema.

- Protection against Chronic Illness: A number of diseases are at risk due to chronic inflammation. Anti-inflammatories may aid in preventing several ailments by lowering inflammation.

Anti-inflammatories may cause negative effects, particularly if taken over an extended length of time. Before using any anti-inflammatory drugs, consult your doctor, particularly if you have any underlying medical issues.

2.3. Impact on Cardiovascular Health

Research on hydrogen gas's possible effects on cardiovascular health is an exciting and quickly developing field. Even though the data so far is encouraging, more thorough and extensive research is required in order to reach firm conclusions and provide specific recommendations.

Hydrogen has anti-inflammatory and antioxidant qualities. It works as a selective antioxidant, destroying damaging hydroxyl radicals while sparing healthy free radicals. This shields cells from oxidative damage, which is a major cause of heart-related illnesses. Furthermore, hydrogen has anti-inflammatory qualities that may lower the risks of cardiovascular inflammation.

Research indicates that hydrogen may offer cardiovascular protection against ischemia-reperfusion damage, a frequent side effect following surgery or organ donation. It may also enhance energy

 Research indicates that hydrogen may enhance endothelial function, which may increase blood flow and thus lower the risk of cardiovascular events

According to scant research, hydrogen may be able to help people with hypertension reduce their blood pressure.

With small-scale clinical trials and pre-clinical investigations, the majority of the research on hydrogen and cardiovascular health is still in its early phases.

To validate the effectiveness and safety of hydrogen treatment for particular cardiovascular disorders, more extensive, long-term trials are required.
Dosage and delivery: It's still uncertain what the best dosage and delivery strategies are for various cardiovascular uses. For safe and efficient practices to be established, more study is required.

Hydrogen shows promise as a possible therapeutic agent, but it might work better when paired with already-approved, scientifically supported cardiovascular medications.

Suggestions:

Speak with your healthcare provider before pursuing any kind of hydrogen therapy for cardiovascular health. Based on your particular situation and medical background, they can offer advice on the possible advantages and disadvantages.

Give lifestyle interventions top priority: Sustain a healthy lifestyle that includes regular exercise, a balanced diet, enough sleep, and stress reduction. These are essential for the best possible cardiovascular health.

Keep up with the most recent findings in the field of hydrogen and cardiovascular health research to learn about the changing perception of this material's possible application

It's exciting to consider hydrogen gas's potential as a useful tool for improving cardiovascular health. It's important to stress, nevertheless, that the state of research today is still very new. It is imperative that you speak with your physician, follow recommended medical procedures, and keep up to date on current research before pursuing hydrogen treatment for cardiovascular health. Recall that although hydrogen has potential as a supplemental strategy, it should never take the place of currently recommended, research-based cardiovascular health practices.

Further discoveries about hydrogen medicine's possible effects on cardiovascular health could be anticipated as the subject develops. Let's welcome the current findings and hold out hope for the potential benefits this innovative

therapeutic agent may have in the future
for maintaining and enhancing heart
health.

2.4. Neuroprotective Benefits

Threats from a variety of sources
continuously target our brains, the
amazing command centers of our

existence. These sensitive organs are susceptible to damage from oxidative stress, inflammation, and neurodegenerative illnesses like Parkinson's and Alzheimer's. Fortunately, antioxidants and anti-inflammatories are strong defenders in our dietary armory, providing promise for safeguarding our neurological health.

Think of extremely reactive chemicals called free radicals as renegade agents that are wreaking havoc on your brain's cells. They cause harm to proteins, DNA, and other important components by stealing electrons. This oxidative stress is linked to neurodegenerative disorders and age-related cognitive impairment.

Another opponent is chronic inflammation, which constantly raises the alarm and interferes with sensitive brain functioning. This internal fire can lead to a variety of neurological diseases by harming neurons and obstructing brain cell communication.

Before they cause damage, these molecular barriers destroy free radicals. Antioxidants maintain cognitive function and shield brain cells from oxidative damage by scavenging these rogue agents.

Among the essential antioxidants that
support the brain are;

- Vitamin C: This strong antioxidant
  helps to keep neurotransmitter levels
  in check and shields neurons from

- Vitamin E, which is present in nuts
  and seeds, protects the membranes of
  brain cells from oxidative stress.

- Flavonoids: Found in dark chocolate
  and berries, these plant-based
  antioxidants enhance cerebral blood
  flow and shield brain neurons from
  harm.

These substances suppress the inflammatory fires inside the brain, much like firemen do. They safeguard neurons and advance a positive mental environment by lowering inflammatory mediators. Key anti-inflammatories that are beneficial to the brain includes:

- Fatty fish contains omega-3 fatty acids, which lower inflammation and support the health of brain cells.

- Curcumin: The active component of turmeric, curcumin has strong anti-inflammatory qualities that shield cerebral tissue.

- Resveratrol: Resveratrol is an antioxidant and anti-inflammatory substance that is present in red wine and grapes and is beneficial to brain health.

The combined impact of antioxidants and anti-inflammatories results in the best possible protection for the brain. By addressing various facets of neurodegeneration, they offer a broader safeguard against cognitive deterioration and neurodegenerative illnesses.

It's important to keep in mind, though, that every antioxidant and anti-inflammatory has a different set of advantages. Some may be more effective than others in focusing on particular brain regions or networks. To best support your brain health, you can customize your food choices and think about possible supplements by speaking with a healthcare provider.

Although these substances have a lot of promises, maintaining a healthy lifestyle is still the key to brain health.

Have a diet high in fruits, vegetables, and
whole grains that is well-balanced.
To increase blood flow to the brain,
engage in regular exercise. Take part in
cerebrally engaging pursuits such as
reading and solving puzzles.
Obtain adequate restful sleep.
Use calming methods to reduce stress,
such as yoga or meditation.

Through the integration of a brain-friendly
diet and way of living with the possible
advantages of antioxidants and anti-
inflammatories, you can develop a
multifaceted strategy to protect your

neurological well-being and prevent cognitive decline for many years to come.

Keep in mind that the brain is a very flexible and robust organ. It is possible to empower your brain to flourish and confidently confront the obstacles of aging and neurodegenerative disorders by being proactive and supplying the necessary resources.

2.5. Detoxification and Immune system Support.

The idea of "detoxification" in order to support the immune system has generated a lot of discussion and misunderstanding. Although the body has complex natural processes for getting rid of waste and toxins, the word "detox" frequently refers to certain diets or exercise routines with conflicting scientific evidence. It's crucial to approach this subject cautiously and comprehend the intricacies of detoxification as well as any possible effects it may have on your immune system.

Effective detoxification processes are already present in our bodies. They are;

- The liver: This serve as the body's main filter, breaking down and digesting toxins before excreting them in the form of bile or urine.
- Kidneys: Remove waste materials from the blood and eliminate them through pee.
- Lungs: You can exhale to get rid of poisons.
- Through bowel movements, the digestive system gets rid of waste and partially digested food.

- Fluids and cellular waste materials
  are drained and filtered from tissues
  by the lymphatic system.

Together, these systems keep us safe and
get rid of potentially dangerous pollutants.

Numerous detox diets and regimens make
the promise to improve the immune
system and accelerate the body's cleansing
process. These frequently entail:

- Restrictive diets: cutting out
  particular food groups (such as dairy,
  meat, sweets), or limiting one's

intake to particular cleanses or juices.

- Following certain liquid-only or fasting regimens, one may refrain from eating for a while.

- Detoxifying products or supplements: encouraging supposedly toxic waste removal

Though there is little scientific evidence to support these techniques' ability to improve immunity and detoxification, they may cause temporary weight loss or alterations in bowel patterns. Concerns over possible electrolyte imbalances and vitamin shortages linked to restrictive diets, particularly when followed for prolonged periods of time, are voiced by certain specialists.

Making a healthy lifestyle a priority provides a more long-lasting and efficient method of immune system support:

- Consume a well-balanced diet, emphasizing fruits, vegetables, whole grains, and lean protein to provide your body the nutrients it needs for optimum immunological function.
- Remain hydrated: Consuming enough water promotes general

health and aids in the removal of pollutants.

- A lack of sleep can impair immunity, so make sure you get plenty of it. Try to get 7–8 hours of good sleep every night.
- Handle stress: Prolonged stress might impair immunity. Use calming methods such as yoga or meditation.
- Engage in regular exercise: Exercise strengthens the immune system and circulation.
- Reducing alcohol and smoking use can help strengthen immunity.

Above all, see your doctor for specific advice before starting any extreme diet plans or detoxification regimens. They can assist you in determining whether these procedures are appropriate for your particular requirements and medical problems.

CHAPTER 3. APPLICATIONS AND PRACTICES OF HYDROGEN MEDICINE

3.1 Inhalation Therapy: Breathing Hydrogen Gas

Inhalation therapy using hydrogen gas (H_2) is a rapidly developing topic in medicine that has great promise for treating a range of medical disorders. Although more study is required, the initial results show promise.

As a selective antioxidant, H_2 protects healthy free radicals from injury while concentrating on the damaging hydroxyl radical (OH·). A major contributing factor to many diseases, oxidative damage, is prevented in healthy cells by using this focused strategy. H_2 also demonstrates anti-inflammatory qualities, which lower the generation of inflammatory mediators and may help with chronic pain and arthritis.

While there are other ways to administer H2 for medicinal purposes, inhalation has the following benefits:

- Direct targeting: Breathed H_2 maximizes its therapeutic benefits by

entering the bloodstream and lungs
fast.

- Non-invasive: Since inhalation doesn't require needles or injections, patients find it to be a more handy and comfortable treatment.

- Control of dosage: Having precise control over the quantity of H2 breathed enables customized treatment.

According to research, H_2 inhalation therapy may be useful in treating a number of illnesses, such as:

- Neurodegenerative diseases: Research indicates that H_2 may shield brain tissue and enhance cognitive performance in those with Parkinson's and Alzheimer's disease.

- injury during surgery or organ transplantation. The preventive actions of H_2 may reduce this damage.

- Metabolic disorders: Diabetes, obesity, and other metabolic disorders are characterized by oxidative stress and chronic inflammation. The potential benefits in managing these illnesses are suggested by H_2's ability to counteract these causes.

- Further health issues: Studies investigating the possible advantages of inhaling H_2 for illnesses such as inflammatory bowel disease, asthma, and chronic fatigue syndrome are now underway.

The use of H2 inhalation therapy to treat a range of illnesses looks promising. Its special abilities as an anti-inflammatory and selective antioxidant provide a fresh method of treating a range of medical conditions. H_3 may turn into a useful weapon in our healthcare toolbox as research advances, offering promise for better health and wellbeing.

3.2 Hydrogen-Enriched Water and Beverages

In recent years, hydrogen-enriched water, also referred to as hydrogen water, and beverages made with hydrogen gas have gained popularity due to their purported health advantages. The real effects of drinking water that has been enhanced with hydrogen and the science supporting these assertions are still up for debate.

Hydrogen-enriched water is just regular water that has been infused with hydrogen gas using a variety of processes, such as electrolysis or diffusion. While some businesses offer tablets or generators to infuse your own water at home, others sell bottled hydrogen water.

Hydrogen-enriched water proponents list a number of possible advantages, such as:

- antioxidant effects: It is thought that H_2 shields cells from oxidative damage by neutralizing dangerous free radicals, which may lower the chance of developing chronic illnesses.

- H_2 may have anti-inflammatory qualities that may lessen inflammation and ease the symptoms of chronic pain and rheumatoid arthritis.

- Enhanced sports performance: Research indicates that H_2 may facilitate muscle regeneration and lessen post-exercise exhaustion.

- Benefits to cognition: Some study indicates that drinking hydrogen-enriched water may enhance memory and cognitive performance.

Although H_3 appears to have potential benefits theoretically, there is currently little scientific data to back up these assertions. There are methodological errors or tiny sample sizes in many studies, which makes it challenging to reach firm conclusions.

Limited investigation: To validate the efficacy and safety of hydrogen-enriched water for different medical diseases, more meticulously planned, extensive clinical trials are required.

Dosage & absorption: It's still unknown how much hydrogen is actually absorbed from drinking water and what the ideal dosage is for possible health advantages.

Cost-effectiveness: Compared to established medical procedures, the cost-effectiveness of bottled hydrogen water and home infusion equipment may be questioned.

Possible side effects: Although hydrogen-enriched water is usually thought to be harmless, certain studies have noted that eating high amounts of the water may cause potential adverse effects such bloating and diarrhea.

Although there isn't enough proof to draw firm conclusions just yet, the prospective advantages of hydrogen-enriched water and beverages are encouraging. A cautious approach is advised, even though it might have intriguing possibilities for future applications in health. Prior to adding hydrogen-enriched water to your routine, concentrate on leading a healthful lifestyle and speak with your physician.

3.3 Hydrogen-Infused Topical Treatments

Hydrogen gas is starting to make an appearance in topical therapies in addition to water and beverages because of its fascinating antioxidant and anti-inflammatory qualities.

In these therapies, hydrogen gas is infused into creams, gels, sprays, or patches.

Proponents of topical hydrogen-infused treatments point out a number of possible advantages for skin health, such as:

- Dermatitis, psoriasis, and eczema are just a few of the skin problems that the anti-inflammatory qualities of this substance may help to relieve.

Topical therapies using hydrogen infusion is still a relatively new field of study.

Pay particular attention to a balanced diet,
enough hydration, and regular skincare
regimens that have been shown to improve
skin health.

While more research is
need to provide conclusive answers,
cautious optimism about this new area
holds promise for creative ways to support

skin health and possibly help with other therapeutic uses.

3.4 Hydrogen-Rich Foods in Adult Nutrition

Certain food groups naturally produce hydrogen during digestion, even though hydrogen gas itself isn't found in food. These hydrogen-rich food groups can be beneficial for general dietary health and can tangentially contribute to advantages related to antioxidants and anti-inflammatory agents, even though the health effects of ingesting hydrogen through food are still being studied.

The following important dietary groups are high in ingredients that produce hydrogen:

Fruits and vegetables: Packed with nutritional fiber, these produce hydrogen as a byproduct when fermented by our gut bacteria. Particularly healthy sources include fruits (such as berries, apples, and pears) and vegetables (such as broccoli, leafy greens, and sweet potatoes).

Whole Grains: Whole grains such as quinoa, brown rice, and oats contain complex carbs that can be fermented to produce fibers that can aid in the creation of hydrogen and possibly improve gut health.

Prebiotic-Dense Foods:

Legumes: Prebiotics are non-digestible fibers that nourish our gut flora and encourage the synthesis of hydrogen and other advantageous byproducts. Beans, lentils, chickpeas, and soybeans are good sources of these fibers.

The prebiotic fibers found in onions and garlic, known as fructooligosaccharides (FOS), encourage the development of good gut bacteria and the synthesis of hydrogen.

Non-Static Starch:

Cool Cooked Potatoes and Rice: After cooking and cooling down, potatoes and rice acquire resistant starch, which is a fiber type that does not break down in the small intestine and instead travels to the colon, where it is fermented by gut bacteria, generating hydrogen and possibly improving gut health.

Moreso, fruits such as bananas and plantains contains prebiotic fibers like as inulin, which may help produce hydrogen and have other prebiotic properties.
Pears and apples: These fruits have a fiber called pectin that microorganisms in the stomach can ferment to produce hydrogen and possibly enhance intestinal health.

Though eating foods high in hydrogen may have a positive indirect impact on health due to their anti-inflammatory and antioxidant qualities, keep in mind that:

To draw firm conclusions, additional research is required on the medicinal effects of hydrogen derived from food, as the field is still in its early stages.

Regardless of hydrogen generation, gut microbiota diversity and general health depend on a balanced diet high in fruits, vegetables, fiber, and whole grains.

To achieve optimum health, it is not advisable to concentrate only on hydrogen-rich foods and ignore other dietary aspects

3.5 Dosage Guidelines and Safety Consideration.

Hydrogen gas is currently used as a medicinal agent without any established safety procedures or dose recommendations that are agreed upon by all parties. Clear recommendations cannot be established until more research is conducted on the efficacy and safety of this treatment for different health conditions.

That being said, the present knowledge is broken down as follows:

- Inhalation: Research on hydrogen inhalation therapy typically uses oxygen and hydrogen concentrations between 0.2% and 2% for periods of 30 to 2 hours. However, the best dose and length of treatment varies based on the specific ailment being treated as well as the needs of each patient.

- Once more, it is unknown what the ideal

dosage and possible therapeutic advantages are.

- Topical therapies: There has been little research done on hydrogen-infused topical therapies, and studies that have been done have frequently used formulations with different hydrogen concentrations and application techniques. Finding safe and efficient dosing for various skin disorders will require more investigation.

- Food-Derived Hydrogen: Eating foods high in fiber and probiotics produces even less hydrogen than drinking water or breathing it in. Although eating these meals is typically safe and good for gut health, the benefits of this cannot be applied to hydrogen therapy dosages.

Before beginning any hydrogen therapy, including topical treatments, enriched water consumption, or inhalation, you should always speak with your physician or other trained healthcare provider. Based on your unique health situation, they can offer advice on the advantages and disadvantages as well as safe measures.

Keep up with the most recent discoveries

in hydrogen treatment research to

comprehend how dose and safety

procedures are becoming understood.

CONCLUSION:

With so many possibilities for improving adult health, hydrogen gas is an exciting new area of study in medicine. Its anti-inflammatory and antioxidant qualities present fascinating potential for treating a range of ailments, from wound healing and skin health to neurological illnesses and chronic pain.

But it's important to approach adult hydrogen medicine from a realistic, well-rounded standpoint. The current situation is summarized as follows:

Initial investigations indicate that hydrogen therapy may have advantages in a variety of contexts, providing optimism for further advancements.

Hydrogen's specific anti-inflammatory and antioxidant characteristics set it apart from other treatments, maybe offering a fresh way to handle some ailments.

Topical treatments, water drinking, and inhalation provide patients with practical and maybe comfortable choices.

In order to conclusively verify the safety and efficacy of hydrogen treatment for a variety of illnesses, more thorough studies are needed as the majority are small-scale.

 More investigation and established standards are required as it is still unclear what the best dosage and delivery strategies are for various applications.

 Although low amounts are currently thought to be safe, more research is needed to fully understand any possible long-term effects and combinations with other drugs.

Adult hydrogen medicine has amazing potential, but there are still a lot of unanswered questions. It's crucial to have

a critical mindset and cautious optimism.
Prioritizing evidence-based procedures,
following up on research updates, and
speaking with medical specialists before
attempting hydrogen therapy in any form
are essential.

Keep yourself informed, work with your
medical specialists, and welcome the
continued investigation into hydrogen as a
possible future tool for improving and
boosting adult health.